I0408400

Survival Guide for Kids:
25 Important Lessons Your Child Should Know In Order To Survive Emergency Situations

Table of Contents

* * *

Introduction: Growing Up with a Mindset for Survival

We are all taught certain things by are parents in order to ensure our survival. When you were a child you may remember your parents telling you to look both ways when you cross the street, even though you may have zoned out such repeated instruction as nothing more than meaningless banter, such skills are vital to your survival.

Likewise, in the world of today, with rising crime, increasing environmental uncertainty, and other factors becoming rapidly unpredictable, you will need to raise your own children to grow up with an alert instinct for their own future. This book serves as a guide to enable them to do just that. No matter what situation your kids may face, whether it is a natural disaster or peer pressure, you have to stay vigilant in order for them to succeed. You must make it a point for them to grow up with a mindset for survival.

Chapter 1: Lessons in Wildlife Danger

Almost all kid's love animals, this is without a doubt. But as much as they want to run up and say hi to the large Canadian goose nesting in their yard, such decisions could lead to tragic results. If have to teach your kids early on how to approach animals. From domestic cats and dogs to the random wildlife that could show up in your neighborhood, this chapter will serve as your guidepost in instructing how to handle each potential wildlife danger. This chapter breaks down some of the wildlife that they will most likely encounter and how they should approach and deal with each category of animals.

Dogs

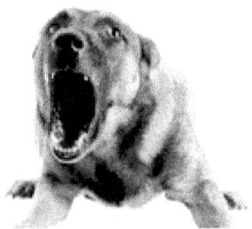

They are man's best friend but if you treat them the wrong way they could turn into a mortal enemy. Often enough children—especially those who have never had pets before—do not know how to approach a dog. Fortunately enough, many dogs are fully patient, long suffering and are fully able to tolerate those that rub them the wrong way. But this isn't always the case, and it only takes one dog to snap, in order for you to have a real problem.

So let's get the basics of dog interaction down form the start in order to avoid these unfortunate situations. Many kids unknowingly scare dogs by excitedly running right up to them and trying to hug them around the neck or otherwise putting their face close to the animal causing the animal to get startled and possibly bite them out of fear. You need to let your child know that the animal needs time to get acquainted with them.

Explain to your child that a dog usually greets another one by sniffing them, and then instruct them to let the dog smell their hand before they attempt to pet them. This way the dog can get used to them and not be too overwhelmed by the interaction. Also inform them never to look the dog in the eyes, since this is a threatening gesture to most animals. Yes, it would seem that us humans are quite the exception, even though with humanity steady eye contact is supposed to demonstrate openness and confidence, for a dog a stare down is a threatening challenge.

So let your kids know not to stare down your puppy! Another big thing that kid need to learn about interaction with their dog, is to never attempt to take anything out of the dog's mouth. While some find it fun to pull on the other end of a chew toy that the dog is munching on, some dogs don't like this, and children often are unable to interpret the cues and body signals from the animal that it is getting angry at being disturbed.

Because of this potential for miscommunication with the animal it is better just to teach your children *not* to take anything away from the dog in the first place. This sort of caution is a good thing, even with household pets, but when it comes to random dogs encountered in the neighborhood, you need to teach your kids to keep their distance.

Tell your children not to approach dog's they don't know. If they see a dog barking behind a neighbor's fence for example, tell them to never put their hand through the fence to pet the dog, this is a dangerous situation since the dog views the yard as its territory, explain to your children that dog's get aggressive when someone they don't know crosses over into their yard. Also inform your kids that a dog that is showing overt signs of aggression such as growling, barring its teeth, or arching its back needs to be avoided at all cost.

And if they see a dog like this out in the open, it is important to *slowly* walk away. Teaching them to slowly extricate themselves fro the situation is important, because the second they run from an aggressive dog, it will most likely just kick in their innate sense to chase after them, which would inevitably lead to a brutal dog attack. So let them know that if they see a dog behaving in an aggressive manner, they need to slowly walk away and find an adult to help them as soon as possible.

Cats

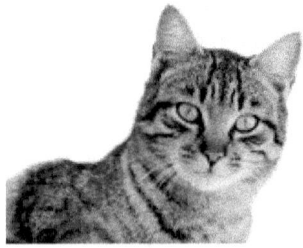

Many parents view the cat as a safer option when compared to the dog but this is largely an erroneous assumption, because even these small animals can become very dangerous if they are provoked. Teach your kids to be careful around the cat if they suddenly see him flatten out his ears, crouch, arch his back up, or begin to emit a low growl. These are all signs to stay away from this agitated animal. Cat's that are agitated will often react to any quick movements, and someone moving quickly past the angry quite is liable to get scratched.

So if you see these signs tell your children to avoid this feisty feline. But besides these emergency measures, you need to instruct the kids not to set off the animal in the first place. Some obvious ways children may agitate a cat is pulling on the animal's fur or his tail. Even the gentlest cat in the world is going to get upset when they are treated like this.

Help your kids understand that their cat is a living breathing creature and not a stuffed animal or toy that they can be rough with. Teach them to be gentle with the animal, to not throw things, and to behave respectfully. Cat's tend to hold grudges, and once it recognizes who it is who is agitating them, they don't forget it very easy. So in order to prevent that cat from sneak attacking the one who has frequently harassed them (it happens), teach them to treat the cat with respect in the first place.

Birds

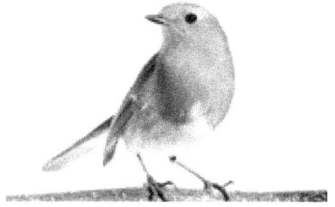

They fly in the air, land in our yards, and we even keep some in cages. Birds are wonderful animals, but they can be dangerous to children if they don't know how to interact with them. Most small bird shouldn't be a problem, but there are some larger birds that can pose a threat.

Many duck species and most especially (as was mentioned at the beginning of this chapter) the ever increasing population of Canadian Geese could pose a hazard. Birds like these are big, sometimes weighing as much as 20 pounds. So when these birds get aggressive and throw all of their weight at you, they can be a force to reckon with. With these kinds of birds, the best policy is avoidance. Teach your children to give these birds a safe distance at all times.

Bees and Wasps

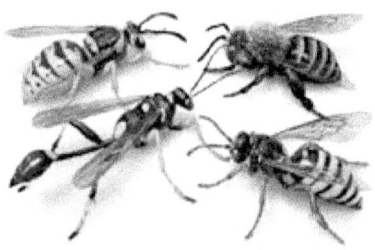

While your child is not as likely to seek out individual bees and wasps as their playmates; children quite often to stumble upon their nests and hives by accident, creating quite a significant danger. Teach your kids to not panic if they are ever stung by bees and wasps. Help them to understand that they need to remain calm and just focus on removing the stinger that bees and wasps have left behind.

They need to especially be careful in this removal because these stingers have a sac full of venom attached to them, and that it is very important to be careful in their removal so that they don't end up squeezing more venom out of the sac. Inform them that they should either wait for an adult, or take a pair of tweezers and use them to slowly pull the stinger out themselves.

Ticks

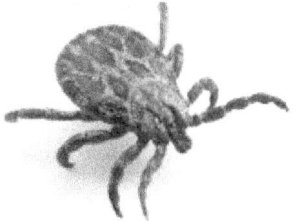

Ticks can be a dangerous critter that your kids might encounter outdoors. These little buggers have the scary habit of burrowing their heads into the skin of those they attach to and become notoriously hard to remove. They hang on as hard as they can while leeching blood out of their host. A soundly unpleasant situation, but you need to have patience in its resolution.

Just like with the removal of a wasp sting, it is best not to panic. Keep your child from trying to scratch, and pick at the tick, it's important not to put too much pressure on the bug or it will lodge itself even deeper. Instruct them to take a pair of tweezers and slowly tug this bad bug out until it falls on the ground. Once the tick is out it can be safely eliminated.

Snakes

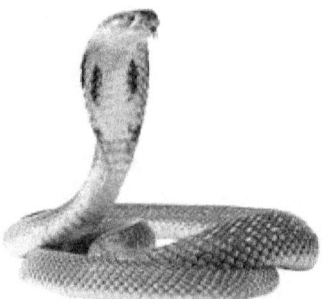

While a snake is not likely to be encountered on a daily basis, they are common enough that there may come a time when they may make their presence known. Having that said, it would be wise to instruct your kids about the danger presented by this form of wildlife. The first thing that should be known when it comes to snakes is that they most likely want to be left alone. Since there is now way a snake could eat a human being, the only reason they would have to strike out and bite you is that they are afraid or thinking they are protecting their territory.

So if you are walking outside and suddenly see a snake in your path just turn around and go the other way. Some of us—especially in western civilization—have such an inborn fear of snakes, as soon as they see them, they wish to kill them. Not only is this a bit unfair for the snake who deserves to live just as much as any other creature, it is also very dangerous. Snakes are lighting fast and many bites occur when someone is attempting to strike the snake with an object.

If you attempt to strike a snake, just be warned that there is a good chance that the snake will see the blow coming and leap in the air to bite you in the arm! This is a very dangerous situation and is best to be avoided altogether. Some snakes have an incredible ability of launching themselves like a missile, propelling forward as much as their whole body length at a target. Having that said, it is important to stay at least 6 feet away from the animal at all times.

If your kids accidentally walk up on a snake, teach them to not make any sudden moves but to slowly walk backwards without letting the snake leave their sight. They can take bigger and bigger steps back as they move away from the animal. They just don't want to do anything to sudden to provoke the animal's attention. Teach your kids caution when dealing with all of these potential dangers in wildlife.

Chapter 2: Lessons in Stranger Danger (Self Defense and Avoidance)

In today's world of crime and unsettling headlines, probably one of the most important survival lessons you can teach your kids is how to avoid and (if needed) protect themselves from strangers. This chapter will highlight some of the best self defense and avoidance practices that anyone can learn in order to stay safe around people they don't know.

Know Where They Are

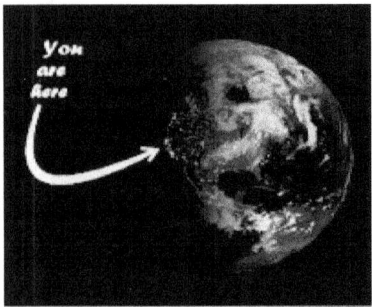

This may seem like common sense. But one of the biggest challenges a child can face is getting lost and losing track of their surroundings. Younger children should of course be under adult supervision, but once a child is old enough to venture on their own, they need to be taught how to know where they are at all times so they don't get lost. Teach your kids to recognize street signs, and if street signs are not available teach them to use landmarks in order to make their way back home.

Teach Children Martial Arts

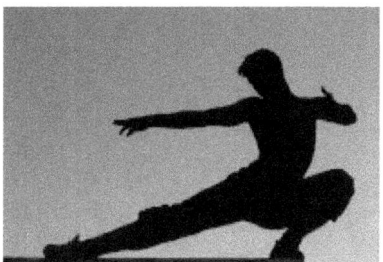

Kids can be trained in basic Martial Arts such as Karate, at a very young age. These classes are good not only for self defense but also for discipline, following instructions and learning responsibility. It is also good to get your kids used to goal setting at a young age, and taking on a course in Martial Arts is a great way to teach them that.

Go for the Shins

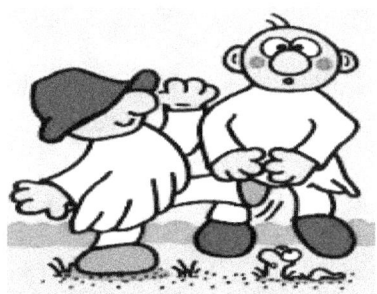

Hopefully your children would never have to face an aggressive stranger. But if they do and someone approaches them, one of the easiest ways to get away, even from someone three times their size, would be for them to kick the aggressor in the shins. If someone is trying to snatch up your kids, a quick kick to the shins would cause the person extreme pain and to stop what they are doing. This would then give your kids plenty of time to run away from the threat that this stranger poses.

Teach Them to Yell for Help

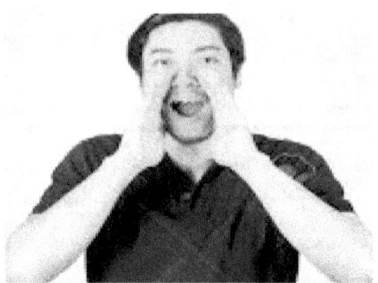

It is important to teach your kids that if someone is trying to accost them, they need to yell and scream as loud as they can to anyone who is around, letting them know that what is happening is not acceptable. If the screaming is raucous enough it should serve two purposes, it should work to alert potential aid in the dangerous situation, and it may very well scare the would-be assailant enough that they change their mind and go the other way.

Don't Talk to Strangers

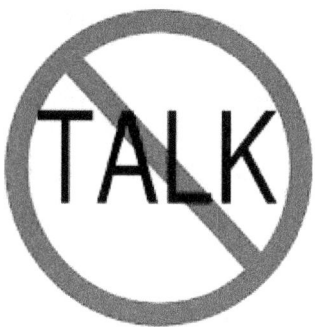

Our final entry in the warnings of stranger danger is of course one of the most common, and something that your own parents probably told you as a child, "Don't talk to strangers". Well, it still holds true today. Teach your kids to avoid excessive conversation with adults they don't know. This doesn't mean that they have to be impolite, or completely unfriendly. If someone politely and respectfully says hello, they can say hi back.

But beyond simple pleasantry of good morning, and hi, how are ya, if an adult attempts to engage in excessive conversation teach your kids to cut off communication. It should be a red flag, especially if the adult is someone that your child does not know, begins to strike up random conversations with a child, most adults—especially in today's world—know not to do this.

So it would be highly unusual to say the least for a random stranger to be that engaged in conversation. Let your kids know to cut these conversations short and simply get away from the person. Just as it was when you were a kid, it still holds true today; don't talk to strangers.

Chapter 3: Lessons in the Dangers of Extreme Weather

Bad weather can strike us anytime and anywhere. And it is especially important that your children know what to do in order to survive the storm. This chapter seeks to inform them of the best lessons they can learn when it comes to weather safety.

Earthquakes

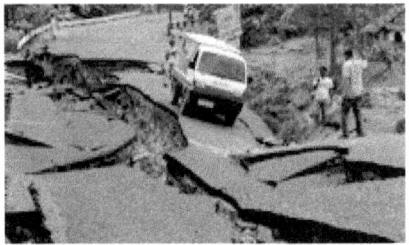

Unless you live in earthquake hotspots such as California, you probably don't take earthquake preparedness very seriously. But if you ask any geologists about the latest trends in the plate tectonics underneath the Earth's crust they would tell you to expect earthquakes to be on the increase in the near future, and that they could strike with little warning in places that previously did not have any history of earthquakes in the past.

Having that said, you should teach your children the basics of earthquake preparedness no matter where they live. Let them know that no matter where they are, if the ground starts to shake they need to head in doors. Whether this means going into school, into a grocery store, wherever, they need to find shelter if a quake starts to break out. Once inside they should find further shelter under a table or desk so that any breaking glass or other falling material does not injure them during the quake. This little bit of preparation could save their life.

Surviving Bad Thunderstorms

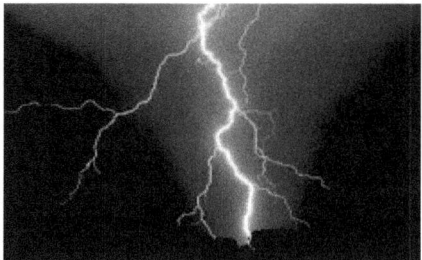

Almost all children are frightened of thunderstorms, and with good reason, lighting can after all cause significant damage and even death. But with the right preparation much of that fear can be alleviated. The number one thing that you should tell your kids when it comes to an imminent storm is to seek shelter immediately. If they are not already inside then they need to go indoors as soon as possible.

If a lighting storm starts when your child is playing in the back yard they may be tempted to take cover under a tree. Since lighting is sometimes drawn to trees, this is very dangerous. Inform them to stay away from trees when a storm hits and go inside right away. Also let them know to avoid water during a storm, if they are swimming a swimming pool when the storm hits let them know of the danger that the possibility of electricity and water poses. Inform them of all of these measures so that you can rest assured that they will survive the storm.

Staying Safe in the Heat

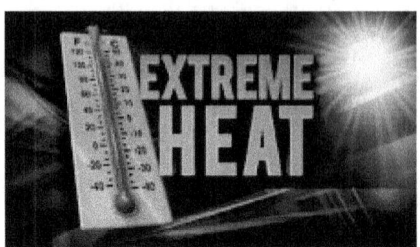

Hot summer days are a good time to play, but if it gets too hot it could pose a significant risk to your kid's safety. Excessive heat can quickly dehydrate the body and raise body temperature to dangerous levels. As a result of this extra stress the heart begins to pump harder in order to bring blood closer to the surface andin an attempt to produce sweat to cool off the body.

But this is only a temporary solution and if relief is not brought soon the body will completely collapse. In order to avoid this teach your children to stay hydrated on hot days, wear loose fitting clothing in which to stay cool, and to immediately go in doors during the hottest time of day in order to avoid becoming overheated.

Winter Weather Safety

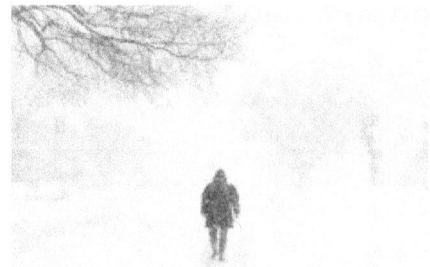

Now that we have talked about how to stay safe in the summer heat, let's talk about how the other side of the weather spectrum and discuss safety during cold and harsh winter weather. Sudden snow and ice storms can hit without warning, and if you are not careful you could find yourself stuck in the melee. You need to especially inform your children of the dangers of "white out" conditions.

A "white out" is in reference to snow storms that bring such rapidly falling snow flakes that nothing can be seen in the immediate area but white snowfall, making it impossible to see even just a few feet in front of you. If your children find themselves in this situation, you need to inform them to stop right where they are, bundle up as much as possible and call for help.

If no help is available they will have to make shelter on the spot and weather the storm. Snow storms often flare up quickly and subside quickly so it is better to stay put and hunker down than to wander off in conditions with low visibility and risk fall through a frozen lake or any number of other dangers. So let your kids know if they are stuck outside in a sudden onset of snow, to bundle up, hunker down, and wait it out!

Hurricane and Tornado Preparedness

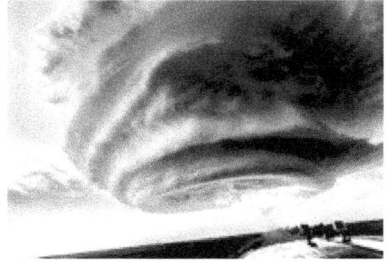

Obviously no one in their right mind would let their children fend for themselves in the face of a hurricane. But even with you right by their side you need to have them ready and knowing what to do without being told. Rehearse with your children ahead of time to stay away from windows and to duck down under desks and tables in order to avoid flying debris if worse comes to worse. Practice makes perfect, so practice hurricane preparedness before that massive storm comes anywhere near your home.

But while a hurricane is an obvious threat that can be seen from a mile away (Most can even be seen from outer space!) tornadoes on the other hand are far more unpredictable and have been known to pop almost out of nowhere. If your child is out riding his bike and a tornado pops into existence, you may not be there to tell them what to do. So in this sense it is even more crucial to explain to them how to handle a sudden twister than it is to weather out a hurricane.

Let them know that if they see a tornado they need to immediately find cover. If there is a ditch nearby tell them to jump into it. Let them know that they can't always assume they can turn the other way and run from the storm. Tell them to find the most immediate structure, whether it is a bridge, a stairwell, or some other structure and hunker down until the tornado passes. Teach them well, and teach them to be prepared!

Surviving Flash Floods

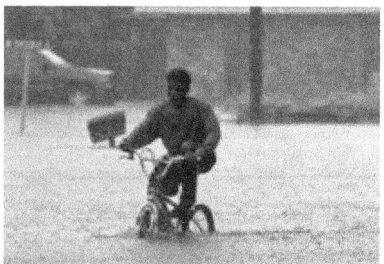

Flooding can be very dangerous, and I am sure you have probably heard the expression, "Turn around don't drown". And it is an important maxim to teach your kids, whether they are attempting to cross a flooded roadway on their bike, or your older teenage children are attempting to cross in their car, you need to make it clear to them that they need to avoid deeply flooded parts of the road.

But beyond road hazards, flash flooding presents the risk of tearing up the very ground itself, sending large rocks and debris in the direction of any pedestrians in the area. But even more deadly is the risk of downed power lines, which can present an invisible hazard, electrifying flood water enough to be lethal. Teach your children to avoid these flood waters at all cost.

Chapter 4: Important Lessons in dealing with Health Hazards

In this chapter we are going to discuss how it is we can deal with health hazards that you're children might face and how to overcome them. A wide variety of possibilities and outcomes are covered detailing the exact means of survival in the given circumstances.

Keeping Kids Safe from Pneumonia

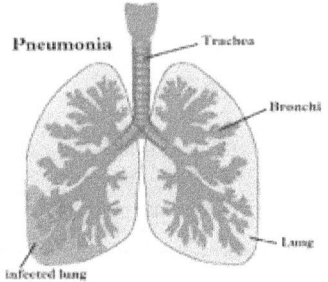

Believe it or not the leading cause of childhood mortality is pneumonia. Many parents don't give it much though, but this is a health hazard that you must protect your children against. Studies have shown that many kids who are susceptible to pneumonia have a zinc deficiency; either from diet or from a biological problem in the absorption of zinc. Make sure that your kids get this precious mineral so that they are not at risk. Also, be aware that pneumonia can be caused by many factors, such as bacteria, viruses or simply extreme cold. Teach your children to be aware of the risks involved in this deadly illness.

Taking Precaution against the Flu

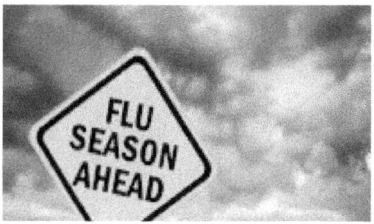

The Flu season hits us every year like clockwork and yet many of us find that we are unprepared. But you really shouldn't let your guard down when it comes to your kids. Make sure they are protected by getting an annual flu shot. It doesn't cost much, even if your insurance doesn't cover it, there are discount programs that can get your child inoculated for as little as $15. It is well worth the trip if it can save your children from contracting the flu.

The Threat of Childhood Obesity

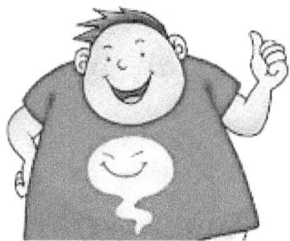

There is a real problem in many developed countries; the problem is childhood obesity. Food is abundant in most households but exercise is not. And as a result we are raising a whole new generation of children who have some major issues controlling their weight. Teach your children early on the basics of calorie management. Teach them exercise and moderation. There is a bad trend towards obesity currently dominating the culture, but you can work now to help your children go against this unhealthy kind of lifestyle.

Diabetes

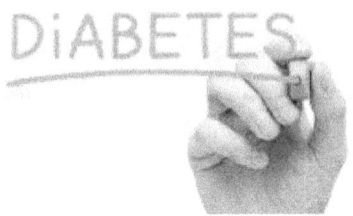

Often related to the obesity epidemic mentioned above, diabetes is becoming more and more common among children. At its heart diabetes is a deficiency in blood sugar levels over a long period of time. One of the major factors aiding in the rise of this health hazard among children is the prevalence of soda and other sugary drinks. Teach your children from a young age to use moderation when comes to drinks and snacks that have high sugar content.

Asthma

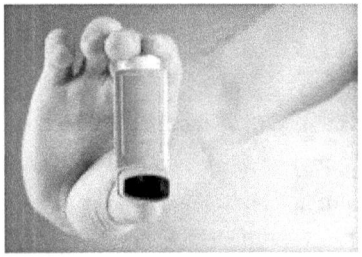

Having asthmatic related difficulties is quite common among children. I can speak about this one from personal experience. And as a childhood asthma sufferer I can attest to the fact that children need to be informed about how to use their asthma inhaler. Asthma is no laughing matter, and can even be deadly in some cases, if you have a child with asthma, teach them to have their inhaler on them at all times.

Allergies

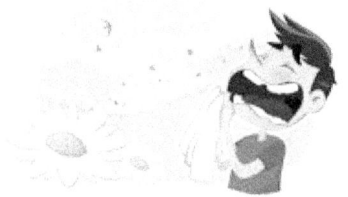

We mentioned asthma, now lets take a look at an illness that is often associated with asthma; allergies. Allergies have risen to absolutely epidemic levels in recent years. Kids seem to be allergic to all kinds of things, from cats to peanuts, there seems to be a high susceptibility to allergic reactions. Have your child checked out early for these kinds of conditions and be sure to keep them aware of their environment (and what's in it) at all times in order to ensure their safety.

Lead Poisoning

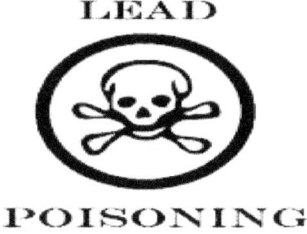

Lead found in the walls of lead painted houses built before 1978 has been a source of great health hazard for children for quite some time. Many kids have gotten sic from picking at the peeling lead paint and putting it in their mouths. If you have young children at home in an old house, you need to especially take caution and let your children know to stay away from this chipping, but deadly lead paint. The hazard of led poisoning rests on a wide spectrum, from death, to causing learning disorders such as attention deficit disorder and memory and speech problems. Be sure to keep your children informed about lead paint poisoning.

Drugs and Alcohol

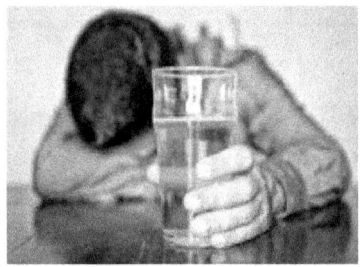

This last health hazard is mostly a warning aimed at older children, because more and more teenagers are getting into trouble from an early onset of drug and alcohol abuse. Kids as young as 13 years old are becoming alcoholics, and drug addicts, in order to counter this trend, parents must take a strong role early on in teaching the dangers of substance abuse.

Children should be directed into healthy after school activities such as music and sports in order to minimize the potential of them engaging in substance abuse after hours. All of the health hazards prevented in this chapter are very serious matters and need to be handled with the utmost care in order to ensure the survival of your children and prevent them from getting into trouble.

Conclusion: Learning to Survive

All parents teach their children survival. Birds teach their offspring how to fly, and fish teach their progeny how to swim, this is a natural instinct of all reproducing creatures. It is no different with human beings; we want our children to do well. But there are many dangers in the world today, many that we ourselves did not have to face when we were children. In the face of such uncertainty we want to know that our children will be safe and secure. I hope this book has helped you in that quest. Thank you for reading!

FREE Bonus Reminder

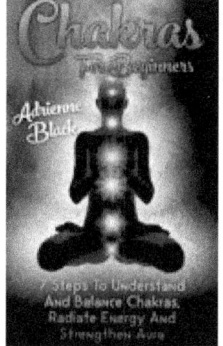

If you have not grabbed it yet, please go ahead and download your special bonus E book *"Chakras for Beginners. 7 Steps To Understand And Balance Chakras, Radiate Energy, And Strengthen Aura"*.

Simply Click the Button Below

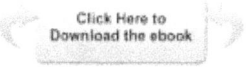

OR Go to This Page

http://lifehacksworld.com/free

BONUS #2: More Free & Discounted Books & Products

Do you want to receive more Free/Discounted Books or Products?

We have a mailing list where we send out our new Books or Products when they go free or with a discount on Amazon. Click on the link below to sign up for Free & Discount Book & Product Promotions.

=> **Sign Up for Free & Discount Book & Product Promotions** <=

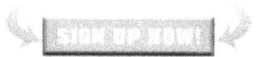

OR Go to this URL

http://zbit.ly/1WBb1Ek

www.ingramcontent.com/pod-product-compliance
Lightning Source LLC
Chambersburg PA
CBHW071322280526
45788CB00004B/1982

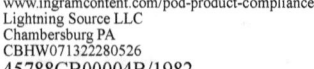